Published By Robert Corbin

@ Hazel Patterson

The Ultimate Dog Training Handbook: A Step-by-step Illustrated Training Guide for Dog Training Success: Better Understanding of Your Dog's Unique Character

All Right RESERVED

ISBN 978-87-94477-06-2

TABLE OF CONTENTS

Chapter 1 1

Dog Psychology 1

Chapter 2 12

Basic Things To Consider Before Starting Puppy Training 12

Chapter 3 21

Puppy Socialization Fundamentals 21

Chapter 4 27

Basic Skills Of Dog Training 27

Chapter 5 41

Bottle Milk And Nutrition For Puppies 41

Chapter 6 47

Puppy Care 47

Chapter 7 56

Physical And Mental Exercises For Your Dog And Breed Selection 56

Chapter 8 67

Basic Dog Care In Adulthood And Seniorhood 67

Chapter 9 107

Resolving A Behavioral Problem In Dogs 107

Chapter 1

Dog Psychology

In order to effectively bond with your new puppy, and have the best relationship possible, a basic knowledge of dog psychology is necessary, and understanding these basics will help you communicate with your dog on a deeper, and more meaningful level. Remember, when you first bring your puppy home, he will be in a strange new place, without his regular pack or littermates. You will have to show your puppy around, and let him know that you will be taking care of him. Be patient, a new home can be scary for anyone.

Dogs need discipline as well as love. They look to their human companion for guidance through consistent discipline and effective training, and can become confused and insecure without that guidance. Your puppy will be safer if you start obedience training early. A well-trained dog can be called away from a potential hazard, and won't chase other people or animals when it is called to heel. Your puppy should also be socialized with other people and animals to be certain that it doesn't become aggressive to, or fearful of strangers and new animals.

How a dog's mind works

Realize that a dog will behave according to its breed. Herding dogs will always enjoy herding something, fishing breeds like to swim. Being aware of your dog's breed qualities will help you understand what instinctual behaviors your dog might be prone to, and can help you satisfy the natural tendencies of your puppy in a healthy, constructive way. This being said, each dog has its own distinct personality, just like humans do.

Dogs have both short-term and long-term memories. They use their long-term memory to remember tricks, like "roll-over" and "sit". Their short-term memory can actually perform better when food is used to reinforce the memory. For a dog, memories are deemed more or less important depending on how helpful they are to their survival, according to their instincts. This is how they can remember that you threw away some bacon in a particular bin, so they will always go back to check that particular bin for bacon! Research has even shown that dogs can dream, possibly, similar to the way that humans do.

Dogs are capable of learning commands, recognition of certain nouns, verbs, and phrases, and can discern the subject matter of a command by following a gaze, or reading the emotion behind your voice. Dogs can also exhibit other aspects of human psychology, such as being susceptible to disorders, like depression or anxiety, and compulsive behaviors. Our canine companions also experience emotions, such as fear, happiness, sadness, and even jealousy. They learn by watching their elders, or other older animals and mimicking rewarded behaviors, and will also mirror emotional cues from their owners in a social setting.

foundation in the changeable, unknown, and sometimes scary world.

Studies show that our dogs love us as much as we love them, our dogs show us in their own ways, too. Some signs that your puppy pair cares for you are:

- Eye contact;
- Wagging tail;
- Snuggling/ cuddling;
- Sleeping with you;
- Bringing you toys;
- Mimicking- i.e. Yawning when you yawn;

Leans against you.

Dogs are the only animals that can intuitively understand human gestures such as pointing. They can understand basic math functions; if they have one treat, and get another treat they know they should have two treats. A dog's cognitive abilities allow it to learn new tricks, remember commands, and figure out just how its human is feeling by studying body language, facial expressions, and tone of voice. Our canine companions are much better at picking up short words and phrases than long ones, and most likely only listen to the first syllable or letter that we say. Dogs use their sense of hearing to process new words. When your puppy hears a new word, they will associate that word with the next new thing in their environment. Once an unfamiliar stimulus, or new word, is detected, the brain switches the learning centers on, in order to understand the new stimulus.

Physical and mental exercise

Now you know that your dog has a mind capable of learning, remembering, and basic problem-solving, but what you may not know is that your dog's mind will work best if you give it some stimulation. Keeping a dog's mind active with mental exercise is just as important as keeping your dog physically active, and there are a number of ways to do this. First, keep your puppy learning. Training your puppy provides him with mental challenges. Training is a mental exercise that can be continued all the way through your dog's life. We wouldn't stop teaching a child to do things after it learned potty training, so why stop training your puppy? Once you have the basics, like sit, stay, and heel, under your belts, keep going. You can find lots of ideas for tricks to teach, or new commands to try, in order to keep your dog engaged in learning. New mental challenges can also keep your dog calmer, by alleviating boredom. Socializing your dog frequently will also provide positive stimuli. When your dog's senses are engaged meeting new people and animals, it will be more alert and better able to handle meeting new people and animals later on.

Dogs learn by repeating behaviors that attain good results, and not repeating behaviors with negative ones. While dogs do experience emotions such as contentment, anger, excitement, and love, experts widely believe they don't feel some of the more complex emotions like guilt and pride, or shame. If a puppy seems to be cowering with guilt and shame next to a mess he just made, it is more likely to be related to the fact that he's equating the mess with punishment, not the fact that he made the mess.

Often, when a dog is having a difficult time picking up new words during training, the human is giving a mixed cue, like lowering the head while giving a command. The dog hears the command to do one thing, but the body language says something else.. When a dog follows a command, they are listening more to the inflection and tone of voice we are putting into that word or phrase when we say it than the actual command itself. Basically, they are reading the intention behind our words, based on the body language, emotional, and vocal cues they are given. This is why you can get a dog to "stand up" or "dance" with a high-pitched, baby-talk voice, but it's much more difficult to get them to calmly sit using the same voice. The best way to keep them calm is if you remain calm yourself, this way your intentions can be read in a relaxed and positive manner. Coupled with an innate desire to please their human companions, a dog's intelligence makes them eager and willing students who want to learn what we have to teach them, and by learning to communicate more effectively with our dogs, we can enrich their minds and train them to become a well-behaved member of the household.

If your dog seems restless, or if you've noticed some breed specific destructive tendencies, you can try and engage them in a game that satisfies their breed instincts. A retriever, for example, will likely be most satisfied playing fetch, and most terriers will like to tunnel. Find creative ways to get your dog doing a job it naturally wants to do. A fun challenge for you and your puppy are interactive games and toys. There are many toys on the market now that allow you to hide a treat inside, so that your dog can solve the puzzle of getting their reward for themselves. Memory and board games are even available, for a fun and exciting way to challenge and engage your dog's mind.

Taking your dog with you as you run errands is also a stimulating experience for your puppy.

Even a short trip to drop off mail, or to pick up some takeout will provide your dog with numerous new smells and experiences, and actually make for a calmer dog when you are finished and return home. Rotate toys to keep your puppy entertained. Once a new toy is brought into the home, Let your dog play with it until they show less interest, then switch it out for either a new toy, or one that they haven't played with in a month or so. Your dog will be just as excited by the toy he hasn't seen in a month, as he will by a brand new one, and they will remain entertained by their toys longer this way.

Puppies need lots of exercise as they grow, and play time is important for your dog's development, health and happiness. Walking your new friend can be a healthy benefit for both you and your pet. Even if you are just walking around your yard, time spent outside just sniffing and exploring is a well-loved treat for your puppy. You can also try keeping some treats handy while walking your puppy, especially if you are still house breaking him. A small reward when "business" is done outside is a powerful incentive for your puppy that he will want to earn again.

Chapter 2

Basic Things To Consider Before Starting Puppy Training

You brought home a new lovely puppy and all the families are happy to see him join the family. The puppy will get lost in the kind of excitement he sees.

Nonetheless, as times go by, he will use the scenario to adapt himself with his family as you took him the first time. But to do that, you need a puppy training methodology to produce this kind of performance. If you like, you can get this sort of technique.

Yet I will give you the best 4 basic techniques.

Too many people have the issue of puppy pooping anywhere in their home. Puppies do not come conditioned with potty and they will do it anywhere they feel like it. This puppy training method will decide how much you will enjoy the puppy and the family.

When you use this form of discipline, please do not use punishment, treat it like your baby. Puppies like it when you notice them rather than recognize them. By commending them, they are going to want to impress you all the time. It is open to children or horses.

You can no longer train your puppies if you allow your puppies to develop into dogs without providing them an appropriate training like this form of puppy training methods, as they mature. These are the simple strategies you can use to succeed.

Well done – you need to recognize when your dog needs to potty. Every puppy has signals when they want to do something about it and wonders about the house. These are the signals they need.

Strong strengthening — this is the basic preparation to be performed. That form of training is the mix of how you teach him to go out and sit and stand, kneel or stuff like that. Be consistent in teaching him to make him understand quickly.

Make sure that your family members engage in the class. Yet you have to remind them to use the term to stop complicating issues. Do not stretch a puppy; let your family member know about it as well. Loyalty is the main word here, as this is what makes them want to know quickly.

Good timing is the easiest thing to do and let your dog know when to do his thing always. Take your puppy out at any point in the morning, when you want him to do his thing. Make sure you have a clear location and time when you feed him.

Taking him out for toilet every half to an hour after he is done feeding him. It helps them to understand their routine and the schedule.

Crate teaching- let him understand the crate's value. Make it clear that the crate is his house if you go shopping or on a break, you can quickly take him there.

Patience is a very important quality of humans. Unfortunately, many of us lack this quality. When it comes to puppy training, this is a vital quality to have in order to achieve the best results.

This is because it will take you a lot of time until you get results with your training and that can be frustrating. Puppy training does not look like a hard task to perform but in reality it is.

The puppy training is an ongoing process. You have to perform it for a long time in order to see the first results. The puppy has to learn what each command means before he can execute it.

You need plenty of time and patience in order to train your puppy into a well-mannered dog. Everything is new for you and your puppy and he might fail to understand your requirements in the first days of training.

If you will not have enough patience and you will become frustrated, chances are your puppy will notice that and think you want to play with him. This will frustrate you even more. If this happens you should definitely call it a day and begin your next training session the next day.

There are some things you can do in order to avoid becoming frustrated. For example, when you feel frustrated you should think that learning new things is hard for people too.

Also, your loving puppy is young and for him is like learning a second language. With efforts on your side and a lot of hard work you will surely manage to train your puppy well.

You should be calm and patient with your puppy because he does not understand your words but he may understand your mood. If you will be upset your puppy will understand that and wanting to cheer you up he might play or roll over.

This will only make the situation worse. So, if you feel you can't be calm, you would better call it a day and continue the puppy training on the next day.

If you lack patience and you feel you can't manage puppy training you may opt for hiring a professional. This way you will enjoy the benefits of having a trained dog as well as not having to work for that.

Another option would be not getting a puppy at all or getting a trained older puppy. If you lack patience, a puppy might not be a good option for you at this moment. This is because patience is needed for training the puppy at least in the first year of his life.

How to Tell If Your Puppy Needs Formal Training

Since owning a marionette is a big responsibility to an owner, one of these duties is to have marionette training as soon as possible. The question here is how to tell if your puppy can be taught by you or whether he wants formal courses.

Some puppies always respond to training quicker, while others still can't master commands, even with the best home trainer. These are the kinds of dogs that will benefit from intensive instruction in obedience. The trainer will targeted your puppy's issues and solve them in his training.

Some dogs just react better to people without even raising a puppy. If you have a puppy that does that, count yourself very lucky because the majority of animals are not like that. This does not mean your puppy is a wild beast. It just means that he is not used to publicly performing properly, and he needs instruction.

Such formal training will teach your puppy the simple obedience commands and how to respond when strangers are around. If you have any issues with your puppy when you carry him home, recommend getting formal instruction.

Another way to determine whether your pet needs intensive puppy training is to decide whether it is on your calendar. Moreover, since it can cost a lot of money, you must also be able to afford the lessons.

If they both don't work out, you don't need preparation. Although it may take longer, it will be the most economical for your family. There is no point in wasting money on anything you can't do for yourself.

If you seek to train your dog alone but cannot conform to a certain timetable, it might be better to attend puppy school. That is because dogs know the most when they are finished on a timetable. When you miss a week or two, your puppy will probably forget where you left off and then start all over again.

When you decide to train your puppy, there are a lot to remember. The most important thing is to determine if it is best for you to do a home training or class and to stick to your plan of choice.

Chapter 3

Puppy Socialization Fundamentals

Allow your puppy to get used to various situations and prepare him for challenges in the future by teaching him fundamental socialization skills. Here are 5 tips and tricks to guide you:

1. Keep things light.

Use the leash to make the social connection. Introduce your puppy to one person or dog/other animal at a time, with the help of his leash for control. Make sure to exercise him to calm him down before any meeting; it also helps to have handy treats to encourage as well as reward your puppy for behaving well. Using a leash will also help you immediately correct him as needed. To make introductions go even more smoothly, act confident around your puppy, and see to it that the visitor is relaxed.

Make sure to give attention to the resident dog by petting him. This will also assure him that everything will be all right with his meeting with your puppy. If things do not go as you hoped they would, it might be better to put off the meeting and introduce them again some other time.

2. Practice damage control, especially when introducing your pup to other dogs.

Make sure your puppy and the dog you are introducing him to are within each other's sight. If introducing your puppy to three or more dogs, let him meet one dog at a time. If you find the animals receiving each other well, don't hesitate to pet, praise, and give a treat to each dog – this shows them that being with each other will allow good things to happen.

Keep an eye on stiffening up, staring, back-fur rising, and other warning signs. Never punish one dog reacting to the other in an aggressive way. It would be better for you to bring him to somewhere he could be alone; allow him to settle down and then ignore him. Do the same with each dog if they both start acting aggressively. You may then introduce them again some other time.

3. Remember that timing is everything.

Timing is important when it comes to correcting any dog behavior that is unacceptable. Avoid waiting for one dog to lunge at the other. As soon as you sense any hint of aggression, immediately correct him by firmly saying "No" as you yank the leash for correction, not punishment. This will bring the aggressor's attention to you and get the message across that you are the leader of the pack. You have no reason to feel alarmed if your puppy does not warm up to other dogs right away; otherwise, especially if this goes on more than one to two weeks, a consultation with a dog specialist may be in order.

It usually takes days or weeks for dogs to acclimatize, so give your puppy about ten to fifteen minutes of daily quality time with you. Play with your dog, give him a massage, brush his coat, and practice different training skills with him. As soon as your puppy reacts well to other dogs, you may then remove their leashes. You will still need to watch over them though, and keep a whistle or spray bottle around to distract them when they start showing aggression. It also helps to have treats on hand for rewarding good behavior.

4. Allow your puppy to ease into the socialization training process.

Your puppy may feel stressed and overwhelmed with surrounding changes, which is why getting him introduced to too many people is not such a good idea. Delay any socialization until your puppy gets settled in his surroundings than risk having him constantly nip or cower whenever he meets other people.

5. Make room for difficulties along the way.

You can expect your puppy to act like one – he will likely growl, jump on people, and engage in other behaviors that need correction. It also helps to ask other people to refrain from playing biting, tug of war, wrestling, or any aggressive game with your dog.

Chapter 4

Basic Skills Of Dog Training

In this section, I focus on some basic skills that your dog needs to know. These are simple skills that are easy to teach and with the same degree of understanding.

Some of these basic skills you need to introduce into your dog training include the following:

Responding to the Clicker

Teaching your dog some commands requires the dog to be familiar with the clicker and respond to it on command. The goal is to let your dog know that it has done something desirable whenever you use the clicker. Take these simple steps to teach it this fundamental skill:

Click the clicker and offer your dog a treat if it responds to the clicking.

Repeat this for a couple of times until your dog gets used to the sound and responds to it.

Naming

Give your dog a name to differentiate it from other dogs in your neighborhood. While that may be simple, you have to teach the dog to respond to the name you give it. This is how to go about the training:

Click the clicker and call the name you want to give your dog.

If it looks at you, you give it a reward.

Repeat this a couple of times and praise the dog whenever it answers you. Do this until the dog can respond to that name without you using the clicker.

Sit and Stand Command

Sitting is one of the simplest skills you can teach your dog. If you can successfully teach a dog to sit, it becomes very easy to manage the dog and gradually teach it some other skills. Follow these tips to successfully teach your dog to obey this simple command:

Get down to the dog's level.

Hold a treat close to the dog.

Gradually raise the treat as you raise your hand.

As the dog follows the treat, his butt will move towards the floor.

When the dog's butt finally touches the floor, give it the treat and praise the dog for doing that.

Don't forget to use the word "sit" as the dog's butt moves towards the floor.

Repeat this training multiple times daily.

You can reverse the process to teach the "stand" command.

Release

- The "Release" command is easy to teach too. These tips will help you achieve that in no time:
- Give your dog a toy and ask it to take it.
- After playing with it for a couple of seconds, hold a treat to the dog.
- When the dog releases the toy, give it the treat.
- Repeat the training and include the "Release" command.
- Repeat the training at intervals until the dog understands and obeys the command.

Come and Stay Command

- These commands are useful if you want to prevent your dog from wandering off or becoming a nuisance. You need a leash to teach your dog these skills. After leashing the dog, follow these steps:
- Let the dog sit in front of you while you have a treat in your hand.
- Try to get the attention of the dog.
- Squat in front of the dog slightly and give the "Come" command after patting your thighs.
- Gently pull the dog towards you with the leash.
- Reward the dog with the treat when it moves towards you.
- Practice this command for about a week and see how your dog responds to the commands.
- You can then practice the command in an enclosure, without the leash, until your dog obeys the command without any hesitation.

Teaching the dog, the "Stay" command is a bit different. Nevertheless, these steps will help you teach that successfully:

- Let the dog sit beside you.
- Put your palm in front of it and issue the command.
- Take a few steps back.
- If the dog moves in response to your movement, move the dog back to its original place and repeat the command.
- Keep repeating the command until the dog does not move as you move away from it.
- Don't forget to reward the dog if he stays.

Heel

- The "Heel" command is used to teach your dog to walk beside you, not behind you nor in front of you, when going for a walk.

- Before teaching your dog this command, it is advisable to teach the "Sit," "Come," and "Stay" commands. This prepares the dog for learning this command that is a bit more advanced. Take these steps to teach it:
- Get a clicker.
- Attach your dog's leash to your waist or belt.
- Keep your clicker and treat in both hands.
- When the dog is moving beside you or at the desired place, give it a treat. You can click your clicker if that's what you use as a form of encouragement.

Take

- You can use this command to inform your dog to pick something up for you. You need the clicker effect here.
- Set one of the dog's favorite toys on the ground.
- Wait until the dog picks it up.

- Click and give it a treat.
- Take the toy from the dog and repeat the command.
- Give it a treat if it picks up the toy.
- Repeat the command several times.

Leave

- This command is useful for your dog to let go of whatever it holds. When it holds an animal or another object, you will find this command useful to stop the dog from harming the animal or destroying the object. Put your dog on a leash when teaching this command and follow these steps:
- Drop the dog's favorite toy or food on the floor in front of the dog.
- The dog will go for the item. Use the "Leave it" command after calling the dog's name.
- Use the leash to restrain the dog too.

- Whenever the dog retreats and looks at you, use the clicker and give it a treat.
- Repeat the process as much as possible and give the dog a treat whenever it retreats after giving it the command.

Bring

- By teaching your dog the "Bring" command, your dog goes beyond being just a mere pet. It will become an assistant on all fours. These tips will work after teaching the "Take it" command:
- With the "Take It" command, ask your dog to take a toy.
- Encourage the dog to come to you with the toy by using the "Come" command.
- If the dog comes to you with the toy, give it a treat.

- Repeat the process a couple of times and introduce the "Bring" command as it masters the act.
- With each bit of progress, give it a treat.
- Drop the toy and walk away from it. Ask the dog to take it and bring it.
- If it obeys, give it a treat and repeat this until it needs no prompting to bring it.

Teachings the Dog Names of Things

- It is helpful if your dog can identify some objects in your home. The "Take it" and "Bring it" commands are ineffective if the dog can't identify the objects to take or bring.
- This is how to teach the command:
- Hold the particular object in your hand.
- Ask the dog to touch it.
- When the dog touches your hand, don't give it a treat.

- If it touches the object, use the clicker and give it a treat.
- Mention the name of the object as you encourage the dog to touch it.
- Repeat the process and call the object's name as you encourage the dog to touch it.

Bell

- You can train your dog to ring a bell for a variety of purposes. For instance, you can teach it to ring the bell whenever it wants to go out instead of spinning around or whining. This is how to teach the dog to use the bell:
- Introduce the bell to your dog by showing it the bell.
- If the dog touches it with its nose, give it a treat.

- Encourage the dog to touch the bell with the "Bell" command.
- Repeat this process until the dog can touch the bell willingly.
- Then hang the bell to the door.
- Ask the dog to touch it by using the "Bell" command.
- If it rings the bell by touching it after giving it the command, give it a treat.
- Repeat this process as much as you consider necessary.
- When going out with the dog, let the dog touch the bell before you open the door.
- Continue the training until the dog can impulsively ring the bell.

Eliminating (toilet training)

- It is better to teach your dog how to eliminate on command rather than spending your time cleaning its mess. Consider doing that with these simple tips:
- Assign a specific spot for this purpose in your yard. This ensures that cleaning up will be easier.
- Take the dog to the spot whenever it wants to eliminate.
- Wait until the dog is through with eliminating and give it a treat after clicking the clicker. The treat may come in a variety of forms. The key is consistent training.
- You can introduce some commands such as "Find a good spot" to encourage the dog to cultivate the habit of eliminating on command.

- Whenever the dog uses the designated spot to eliminate after being issued the command, give it a treat.
- These are the basic skills that your dog must know before you get into some advanced skills. When the dog has mastered them, it will be easier for you to move to teaching it some physical skills.
- There are some physical skills you should include in the list of valuable skills that you want your dog to possess. Let's look at some of them.

Chapter 5

Bottle Milk And Nutrition For Puppies

During the first few weeks of life, a puppy's primary activities are feeding, keeping warm and developing social skills. In most cases, humans will simply watch the mother dog provide all necessary care for her puppies. However, if the puppy in your care has been separated from his mother, or if the mother dog has rejected her young or cannot produce enough milk, caring for the pup is up to you. If you're responsible for taking care of puppies in the first few months of their lives you need to know what milk to use and how often to feed them. Puppies will drink milk from weeks zero to week four, then they will slowly transition from milk to solid puppy food at around five to eight weeks. So, in total, you will bottle feed them for eight weeks. This process of moving them to solid food is known as weaning, which we will cover in the next chapter. Puppies that are still with their mother are easier to take care of as the mother will milk them until she cannot produce any more milk and then she will naturally and gradually stop them from breast feeding and offer them other sources of food. For domesticated dogs, they will transition to solid food such as formulated puppy food or gruel, which is soft or mushy semi-solid food.

What are the puppies' milk requirements for the first four weeks?

- If you own the newborn puppy and its mother is there you should have nothing to worry about when it comes to feeding them. Their mother's milk provides 100 percent of the nutritional needs and you don't have to give them dog food until after the first four weeks of life.

- If the mother dog becomes sick, cannot produce enough milk, or the puppies are found as orphans, you may use a milk replacement.
- When feeding the puppy for the first time, up to two weeks, hold the syringe or teat close to the puppy's mouth and she will instinctively start feeding.
- NEVER feed the puppy on her back or with her head held high, her posture is very important and she should be resting or lying belly down with the bottle or syringe straight in front of her. Having her head tilted too high can cause aspiration which is the inhalation of the formula into the lungs, which can be highly damaging and even fatal.
- During the first weeks of life a puppy's body weight may double or even triple. This rapid

growth will continue, albeit at a decreasing rate, until maturity. Copious amounts of energy and nutrients are required in balanced quantities to support this spectacular growth spirt so feed the puppy often.

- Puppies both need and use copious amounts of energy as you are probably aware from the fact that they start to not sit still and start chasing things and interacting with the objects around them. They need energy about two to three times that of an adult dog which they will get from their formulated milk. Puppies also need about 30 percent of their total energy from protein. Make sure the milk you offer is specifically formulated for puppies. Regular milk isn't catered towards your puppy's high energy needs and may not sit well in your kitty's stomach and cause diarrhea. Your pet will need to eat puppy-formula milk until she reaches maturity.

- Formulated milk and bottles can be bought from pet stores, vets or online and they all have information on how to use them and what ages of the puppy they are suitable for. Milk replacement or formulated milk comes in tubs or drums and is a dry powder or liquid. Follow the instructions on the packet on how many scoops to use and how much water to mix if needed. Puppies need warm milk so there will be instructions on how to heat the milk, usually placing the bottle in hot or warm water. Make sure the milk is lukewarm or body temperature and not hot before feeding. The amount of milk to feed the puppy per day should be on the instructions of the formulated milk.
- Make sure the puppy is warm when they are feeding. You can wrap her up in a small towel or blanket and make sure you are sitting

comfortably yourself as you will have to be patient while your little furball feeds.

Chapter 6

Puppy Care

When purchasing a Cocker Spaniel both first time owners and veteran owners normally opt for buying a puppy. Purchasing a puppy will allow you to establish a good and healthy relationship with your dog and will set the foundation for a long happy friendship. Another reason puppies are so popular is due to the fact that they are among some of the most adorable creatures on the planet! However caring for a new puppy is not the easiest thing. You will have to be prepared to make some huge lifestyles changes to accommodate your new puppy. The following section is a simple and concise guide to help you care for the new canine addition to your family.

Find a Good Vet

Before purchasing your puppy it is a good idea to research the vets in your local area. It is very important to find a vet that is local and highly qualified. The best way to find a good vet is by asking your friends, local dog walkers, local dog groomers, asking the breeder and researching online.

Once you purchase your new puppy you should take it straight to your vet for a checkup. The checkup visit will make sure that your puppy is in good health and free from any serious birth defects or genetic health issues. Introducing your vet to your new Cocker Spaniel while it is young also allows for your puppy to become familiar with the vet – this can help avoid stress during later visits. By taking your puppy to the vet straight away, it also allows you to start a health care routine with your pet. It is important to set up a vaccination plan with your vet and also to discuss the best methods for control parasites (both internal and external).

Food

It is important to purchase food that is formulated specifically for puppies. A decent brand will have a statement from the Association of American Feed Control Officials (AAFCO), or your countries equivalent, on the packaging to ensure that the food you are purchasing is going to fulfil your puppy's nutritional requirements. Small and medium-sized breeds can start eating adult dog food when they are between 9 and 12 months of age. Larger breeds of dog should be fed on puppy kibbles until they reach 2 years of age. It is important to make sure that your puppy has cool, fresh and clean water available to them at all times.

Feeding schedule

Puppies have a different feeding schedule to adult dogs. Their feeding schedule changes as they get older. I recommend feeding your puppy on the following schedule:

- 6 – 12 weeks old: 4 meals per day
- 3 – 6 months old: 3 meals per day
- 6 – 12 months old: 2 meals per day

Obedience training

It is important to train your new puppy to be obedient. Obedience will allow your puppy to have a life full of positive interactions as well as forging a stronger bond between you and your pet. It is important to teach your puppy simple commands such as sit, stay, down and come. These commands will help to keep your dog safe and under control in any potentially dangerous situations. I recommend attending a local obedience training class. Obedience classes allow for you and your dog to learn the best methods for each process and command. Obedience classes also allow you, and your puppy, to interact with other people and dogs of all ages and from all backgrounds. It is important to remember that positive reinforcement has been proven to be a dramatically more effective process than punishment.

Bathroom training

Housetraining is a priority if you want to keep your house clean! Before you start your housetraining it is important to locate a suitable location for your puppy to go to the bathroom. If your puppy has not had all of its vaccinations it is important to find a bathroom that is inaccessible to other animals. This will help to avoid your puppy getting any unnecessary viruses or diseases. There are three key tricks to keep in mind when you are attempting to housetrain your puppy: positive reinforcement, planning and patience. It is important positively praise your puppy when they go to the bathroom outside and not to punish them when inevitable accidents will happen. I recommend the following times to try and introduce your puppy to a bathroom routine:

- When you first wake up.
- When your puppy wakes up from any naps it might have.
- During and after physical exercise.
- After your puppy eats or drinks a lot of water.
- Immediately before bed time.

Be social

The main way to avoid your puppy developing behavioral problems is to be social with it. At approximately 2 to 4 months old, most puppies will begin to accept other animals, people, places and experiences.

It is important to start socializing your puppy with as many people and animals as possible. I recommend bringing your puppy to a dog park, to your friends or relatives houses, to dog friendly restaurants and to have other people accompany you while you walk your pet. By interacting with multiple different types of people and animals your puppy will learn to be more social and accepting.

Signs of Illness

It is important to watch your puppy closely to make sure that it is not exhibiting any signs of illness. Your puppy is at its most vulnerable stage of its development while also being at its most important stage of development. If you notice any of the following signs you should take your puppy to the vet immediately: lack of appetite, vomiting, lack of weight gain, lack of growth, diarrhea, pale gums, nasal discharge, inability to pass urine and stool, lethargy, swelling and difficulty breathing.

Spaying and Neutering

There are a lot of factors to considered when deciding if you should spay or neuter your puppy. Many owners refuse to spay or neuter their puppy due to the fact that they find it morally wrong and unnatural. However most owners do decide to have their pet neutered. Shelter euthanasia is the number one killer of dogs and companion animals throughout America. In Atlanta alone over 15 million dollars is spent annually on euthanizing unwanted dogs! The only way to avoid this is to have your pet spayed or neutered. Dogs face some discomfort if they are in heat or are unable to mate. Spaying and neutering creates no long term health problems for your pet. At the end of the day it is an important decision for you and your family to make. I advise talking it over with your vet and family/friends who have already been through the process.

Chapter 7

Physical And Mental Exercises For Your Dog And Breed Selection

Games to Exercise Your Dog's Body and Mind

As of late, an understudy came to class griping that she had taken her two-year-old Labrador Retriever for a three-mile run, at that point left to get her child from school, and when she got back she found that her pooch had destroyed two love seat pads and was really busy biting the leg off her kitchen seat. That equivalent week, another understudy deplored that when she returned home from the market in the wake of completing an effective 30-minute instructional meeting with her Rottweiler, she found that he had torn up his new case tangle, at that point pulled the curtains off the window and into his case, and was tearing them to pieces. So what was the issue? Shouldn't the Labrador have been physically depleted and the Rottweiler intellectually depleted? Truly and yes. Be that as it may, the way to progress is in destroying them both physically and intellectually. Everything necessary is a bit of arranging. Start with playing these two games, and afterward have a go at making up your very own portion.

1. Wild sits

The most effective method to play: Taught when a canine comprehends the idea of "sit," Wild Sits starts by having the pooch on chain while the proprietor goes around cheering, bouncing all over, and getting the canine irritated up. (Note: If a pooch is docile, apprehensive, or touchy, mitigate the ferocity. The objective is an energized, not alarmed pooch.) Then, mid-cavort, the proprietor will teach the canine to sit. (This should be possible with a treat if the pooch is a pup or new to preparing.) He most likely won't comply with the first run through or two, however after a little practice, he'll have the option to go from acting hyper to sitting quietly on direction.

The advantages: Besides the cardio exercise you and your pooch are getting during this activity, you're showing your canine to hear you out while he's in a condition of hyperactivity. How regularly has your canine gone crazy when the doorbell rings or when he sees individuals in the city and disregarded your arguing for him to sit? Presently you're showing him how to pull himself once more into a responsive and submissive perspective. How extraordinary is that?

2. Cardio twist

Step by step instructions to play: Those who know about the game of deftness realize this activity as weave shafts, however any canine proprietor can show her pet to do it as an approach to have some good times, chip away at coordination, and get a cardio exercise. Essentially set up "shafts" utilizing collapsing seats, orange cones, unused latrine uncloggers, or even individuals, and educate your canine to heel close by you as you weave between them, changing your pace from quick to slow. Consider it being like a slalom course in skiing.

The advantages: Your canine needs to focus more diligently on tailing you as you rapidly alter course. Additionally, on the grounds that he'll remain at your left side as you rapidly weave left and right, he'll need to alter his pace to be increasingly slow, separately, which is the thing that your fitness coach would call interim preparing. Include considerably all the more an exercise by running the whole course.

Give exchanging a shot one of your ordinary instructional courses with these games.

Notwithstanding having a well-prepared and well-practiced pooch, you will likewise receive the rewards of getting more cardio. And keeping in mind that I'm not proposing this can be an option in contrast to heading off to the recreational center, I am talking as a matter of fact that by doing this, your association with your pooch and with your own physicality will improve significantly.

Enhancing your dog's life

Weariness and abundance vitality are two normal explanations behind conduct issues in hounds. This bodes well since they're intended to have dynamic existences. Wild canines spend about 80% of their waking hours chasing and rummaging for nourishment. Residential canines have been aiding and working nearby us for a great many years, and most are reproduced for a particular reason, for example, chasing, cultivating or security. For instance, retrievers and pointers were reared to find and bring game and water fowls. Fragrance dogs, similar to coonhounds and beagles, were reproduced to discover bunnies, foxes and other little prey. Canines like German shepherds, collies, steers mutts and sheepdogs were reproduced to group domesticated animals. Regardless of whether canines were working for us or rummaging alone, their endurance once relied upon heaps of activity and critical thinking.

Today that is altogether changed. Presently the most well-known set of working responsibilities for hounds is Couch Potato! While we're away at work throughout the day, they rest. Also, when we get back home, we serve them free nourishment in a bowl"no exertion required from them. They eat a bigger number of calories than they can utilize. The outcome is hounds who are exhausted senseless, frequently overweight and have an excess of vitality. It's an ideal formula for conduct issues.

What does your dog need?

It's not important to leave your place of employment, take up duck chasing or get yourself a lot of sheep to keep your canine out of difficulty. Be that as it may, we urge you to discover approaches to practice her cerebrum and body. Peruse on for some fun, down to earth approaches to enhance your pooch's life, both when you're near and when you're most certainly not. You'll see that these thoughts go far toward keeping your pooch glad and simpler to live with. Evaluate a couple and see what you and your canine appreciate most.

Tips for Alone Time

Since we as a whole have occupied existences, our pooches regularly wind up spending a decent part of their day home alone. In the event that you give your canine "occupations" to do when she's without anyone else's input, she'll be more averse to think of her own particular manners to involve her time, such as unstuffing your sofa, assaulting the garbage or biting on your preferred pair of shoes. Furthermore, she'll be more averse to energetically handle you when you get back home, after she's gone through a day sitting idle however energizing her batteries!

Getting your puppy the exercise he or she needs

So what amount does practice does your canine genuinely need? There's no solid answer, however enough exercise to feel really worn out.

Most solid pooches will profit by practice sessions in both the morning and the night. A safe, fenced region for off-chain practice is perfect, yet on the off chance that you don't approach this, snap a rope on your little guy and take a walk.

Except if your canine has an ailment requiring constrained exercise, at that point make at any rate one of your pooch's trips a vigorous action. Playing with different pooches off-rope in a fenced zone, swimming, playing bring or running adjacent to a jogger are altogether amazing oxygen consuming activities. Continuously make certain to watch out for your puppy to look for exhaustion and ensure your pooch approaches cool water and shade whenever they are working out.

A few people even train their mutts to run on a treadmill. You can begin with only a couple of moments, and step by step work up to a brief treadmill practice session. Exercise of this nature will discharge endorphins which will have a general quieting impact on your pooch's conduct, just as numerous other medical advantages.

Little dog Safe Activities

Exercises appropriate for grown-up canines may not be alright for developing young doggies. Playing is the best decision for a more youthful puppy, regardless of whether it's off-chain with different canines, playing get or different games with their human. Set up play dates with companions so your little guy can learn social abilities and get some activity.

Running or biking on asphalt are undependable activities for youthful mutts whose bones are not full fledged. If you have any inquiries concerning whether a specific sort of activity is alright for your doggy, check with your veterinarian. Continuously check with your veterinarian.

Remember mental incitement! Instructional courses keep a canine's mind sharp, just as they help create and reinforce the bond among pooch and human. Abstain from exhausting or dreary exercises. Make it fun! Work on instructing your canine stunts like sit and remain alongside basic spryness works out. Short instructional courses are ideal, mixed with play or rest sessions and bunches of acclaim and love.

Chapter 8

Basic Dog Care In Adulthood And Seniorhood

Understanding how to take care of your adult dog is extremely important. If you have owned a dog before, you should know that different stages of its life may require different feeding schedules, amounts, and different types of dog food. An example would be that puppies require puppy specific food that gives them the extra nutrients they need to grow up healthily. Adult dogs don't require nutrient-rich food as that would encourage weight gain. Senior dogs are more sensitive in the sense that they need a specially balanced type of food to ensure they are getting the specific nutrients that they need at an older age while preventing weight gain.

In this chapter, we will be focusing on five elements of basic adolescent dog care. You will be learning about nutrition, hygiene, dental care, neutering, and socialization of your adult dog. We will wrap up this chapter by learning about specific senior dog-related care as it is important to know as well. Just like humans, dogs require different types of diets and nutrition as they grow up, go through puberty, and grow old.

Nutrition

If you have ever gone to any type of pet store or your local department store, you may have noticed the endless aisles of different types of pet food. As a new dog owner, you will be easily overwhelmed by the different options and types of specialized dog foods. Back in the day, the options of dog food were much more limited compared to the present day where endless types of dog foods have been developed due to more advanced research.

Although the process of buying dog food is more difficult now due to the increasing amount of options, it is actually a really good thing for our dogs. Due to the many years of research in the dog food industry, scientists have discovered better ingredients, newer sourcing, and new diet formulas that help increase the overall health of our dogs, puppies, and senior dogs. Unlike the past, we are now able to find all types of specialized dog food like diabetic or diet food in our local pet store. By learning about the necessary nutrients and calories needed for your dog, you will have a better idea of what types of dog food will be able to meet those criteria.

What Type of Dog Food Should I Buy?

As we just discussed, there is such a large variety of dog food available to purchase in the present day. How do we choose which brand to buy? For starters, there are generic types of dog food brands and premium type foods. The premium dog food brands generally offer a higher nutritional density so you are able to feed your dog less but achieve the same nutritional requirements. One major benefit of premium dog food is that their ingredients tend to be stable and does not vary much from batch to batch. Generic dog food brands are less strict on their ingredient compositions so each batch may be different.

Premium dog food companies are big investors in the nutritional research and product development department. They are always looking for innovative ways to upgrade their recipes, formulas, and cutting edge technologies. Premium dog food is a good option for the owners who want to stay on top of the industry and provide the healthiest option for their dog.

However, this doesn't mean you should automatically buy any type of premium dog food out there. Dog owners are actually recommended to take their research one step further by researching and visiting the companies that make their dog food. A lot of the times, your local premium dog food company will offer tours or open houses of their factory and will give you a first-hand look into what goes into their products, how it's made, and where their ingredients come from. My personal recommendation is to choose the premium brands if you have the resources to do so. Typically, the premium brands use high-quality ingredients like premium cuts of meat or organic grains to make their food. Generic brands use more low-quality ingredients like leftover scraps of mixed meat or not pesticide-free ingredients.

To make sure you are keeping your adult or senior dog healthy and happy, you have to make sure that their diet includes 37 specific nutrients. These nutrients all have to be intricately balanced across carbohydrates, proteins, vitamins, minerals, and fats and oils. You may have also noticed that there are different textures that dog food typically comes in. The differences are very large, so it is important to know which type is what. There are three types of dog food that you could serve to your dog. This includes:

Kibble: This is a 100% dry food and the most common type of dog food found. It is more economical compared to the other two types of dog food and provides a complete balanced diet for dogs that come in all breeds, sizes, and ages. This is the recommended type of food for adult dogs as it helps keep their teeth and digestion system healthy.

Canned food: This is a wet food that normally comes in the form of a can. It is the most expensive type of pet food but dogs typically find this type to be the tastiest. Canned food is great for puppies that have not developed the teeth to chew up kibble properly or good for senior dogs that have weaker teeth and digestion. Since canned food is the most expensive type of food, most dog owners reserve them as a treat or on an as-needed basis.

Semi-moist food: This type of food usually comes in single-serving packets and is not a very common type of food. Semi-moist food is not economical and serves very little purpose. This type of food is usually just used as a special treat for their dog.

Experienced dog owners and veterinarians recommend feeding your dog kibble as it is the most beneficial out of all three types, especially if your dog is in its adulthood. It hard texture creates the necessary friction in your dog's mouth when they chew that helps keep their teeth and gums healthy. If your dog is having trouble chewing up the hard kibble, you can add some water into the kibble to help soften it up. You can also decide to mix in some wet food with dry kibble to soften the texture. However, hard kibble without water is the best type of food to feed your adult dog as it is very effective in maintaining good dental hygiene.

Adult dog feeding basics

Since breed, size, age, lifestyle, and health are all factors that play a role in how and what to feed your dog, it is important to consider all of them before purchasing dog food. For example, smaller breeds of dogs tend to have faster metabolisms.

This means that they burn energy and calories at a higher rate. Depending on the specific dog and activity level, some dogs may even need to be fed twice the amount of calories than recommended. The best food formulas for smaller breeds are the ones that contain extra protein and are rich in carbohydrates and fats. This will be the nutrients that will give them the extra energy boost that they require. These types of food also come in smaller kibble size to match the smaller mouths and stomachs of the smaller breeds.

On the contrary, larger breeds tend to have slower metabolisms but they also have bigger appetites! They tend to make larger kibble sizes for large breed formulas to encourage the dog to chew for longer rather than inhaling their food. This type of dog formula has reduced fat and more concentrated protein to prevent weight gain.

Once you have identified the ideal dog food that suits your dog's breed, age, size, and health you faced with the next challenge: how much do I feed my dog and how many times per day? One of the most important parts to making sure your dog is healthy is feeding them the right amount of food. Too little or too much can cause a dog to suffer from nutritional deficiency and obesity-related health issues. Since each dog is dramatically different, there is no easy way to figure out how much a dog should be eating. When in doubt, always consult your veterinarian to make sure that the type and amount that you're feeding your dog is optimal. To give you a basic idea, I have included a recommended daily feeding chart for adult dogs that focus on four different breed sizes; toy, small, medium and large.

Recommended daily feeding for adult dogs

These numbers are based on the total amount of calories that you should be feeding your dog over a 24 hour period. Most adult dogs are recommended to eat two meals a day, so you will need to divide the feeding amount by two and feed that amount twice a day. Make sure you are altering the amount you are feeding your dog based on your dog's lifestyle and their tendency for weight gain. Check your dog's weight every 2 - 4 weeks to keep track of whether they are losing weight or gaining weight. Then, adjust your portion sizes based on your results. Adult dogs who have a healthy weight typically have these traits:

- They have an hourglass figure when they are looked at from above. Their abdomen area should be narrower than their chest and hips.

- They look 'tucked up' from the side view. In other words, your dog's chest is lower to the ground than its belly when standing
- They have ribs that are not easily visible but can be felt with light pressure.

- To help you understand how to determine what type of food and how much of it to feed, I will provide you with two examples.

Hygiene

As we all know, some dogs are smellier and dirtier than others. Although humans don't expect dogs to be clean and good smelling all the time, it is important to make sure your dog isn't so bad smelling that people have to hold their breath. Keep in mind that there is more to dog hygiene than just giving your dog a bath. Dental hygiene is extremely important in adult dogs as that is the prime time when they can develop many diseases or even tooth rot. In this chapter, we will be exploring the importance and techniques for general hygiene and doggy dental care.

Bathing your dog

A common mistake that dog owners tend to make is over bathing their dogs. This is simply due to the mindset of not wanting a 'dirty' dog in your home lying on your bed or furniture. However, dogs don't actually need to be bathed often. The oils in their skin are essential to your dog's skin overall skin health. If you over-bathe your dog you may cause skin conditions for your dog such as dandruff. Veterinarians recommend dogs to be bathed once every three months. If your dog has long hair or is more active, it is appropriate to bathe your dog more frequently.

It is also important to learn where and how to bathe your dog properly. If you have a dog that is of a smaller breed, you are able to wash them conveniently in your sink or bathtub. If you have a larger breed you would have to opt for a larger space where you have access to water. Unlike puppies, larger dogs are harder to restrain especially if they don't enjoy baths. Make sure you choose an area where you have plenty of space and access to warm water. Most pet stores will actually have a free dog washing area where anyone can come in and wash their dog. These places will have removable nozzles that you can use to spray down your dog effectively and also supplies warm water. You should never bathe your dog in cold water as their skin is quite sensitive and would cause irritation that may prevent them from being warm.

Having a well-trained dog is super useful during bath time as you can simply use commands to get them to stay still. If you have an adult dog that does not know the simple commands, make sure you have taught them these commands in order to make bath time less of a battle. In order to prevent you from going into a bath situation unprepared, consider these tips below:

- Before you begin the bath, brush your dog's hair or fur with a brush. Make sure that there isn't any matted hair because matted hair holds a lot of water. It will be difficult to dry and be painful in the washing process. If you can't brush or cut out those mats before the bath, take your dog to a professional groomer instead. Do not attempt to get rid of any mats if you are not confident. Before you begin the bath, make sure to put a large cotton ball in your dog's ear to help keep out the water.

Water in your dog's ear increases the risk of ear infections.

- Make sure you always use lukewarm water to bathe your dog. The water should never be hot but just warm enough where it is comfortable. Keep the water even cooler if your dog is a larger breed as they tend to heat more easily.
- Talk to your dog in a calm manner during the bath. Dogs can become irritated and misbehave during this time, try to soothe their nerves by speaking gently. Make sure to get into a routine of taking baths every few months so your dog can get used to this process and it will feel less foreign to them. Especially if your dog is in its adolescence, they may not have experienced bath time before so easing into it will be more effective.
- Always use shampoo specialized for dogs to bathe your dog. Dog shampoo is made to dry

out skin much less than human shampoo. Use the shampoo once your dog is completely wet and lather it into your dog's body and give your dog a gentle massage. Be sure to avoid their eye area as it could irritate their eyes.
- Rinse out your dog very well after shampooing. Make sure there are no more soap suds left in your dog's fur. Leftover shampoo in your dog's fur can cause skin irritations.
- Let your dog shake out the excess water after the bath (beware, you may get soaked too!). Then, air dry your dog after the bath. Avoid using appliances like blow dryers as it tends to be too warm for your dog's skin. However, there are blow dryers that are made for dogs that you can purchase. This type of blow dryer expels air at lower temperatures to avoid irritation.

- Make sure to reward your dog with a treat after the bath. After the bath give your dog lots of praise. This will help your dog have a positive association with bath time and make them less irritable in the future. This is especially important if you have adopted an adult dog that you're not sure if they have been given baths before.

If your adult dog is particularly irritable and misbehaved during bathtime, you may opt to take them to a professional groomer instead. Instead of going through a strenuous struggle with your pooch, dog groomers are trained and have the equipment needed to properly restrain your dog during this process. Groomers also go the extra mile and help trim your dog's nails, clean their buttocks area, and clean difficult areas like their ears. Most dog groomers are priced very reasonably and do such a thorough job so you don't have to take your dog again for a few months.

Since adult dogs are typically larger and stronger than puppies, they are a lot more difficult to restrain during bath time. As mentioned earlier, make sure that your dog knows simple commands such as 'sit', 'stay', or 'down' before engaging in bath time. Having some way to restrain and command your dog will make bath time more manageable. If your dog is a senior dog, be careful to not be too rough during bath time as they are more prone to anxiety. Make sure to be extra gentle and make the process as quick as possible.

Dental care for dogs

The most common disease for adult dogs is gum disease. Surprising right? Most people think that it would be something like heartworms or cancer but the most commonly reported illness is gum disease. This is usually due to the infrequent dental cleanings that we give our dog. Since gum disease is caused by the buildup of tartar on teeth, if your dog's teeth aren't being cleaned often enough, the tartar can cause bacterial infections in the teeth and gums which can be very lethal. The simplest way to avoid this disease is to brush your dog's teeth every day. This is especially important in adult dogs as they have already lost their baby teeth and are onto their last permanent set of teeth.

Normally dog owners will use a toothbrush made for dogs to do the teeth cleaning. However, if you don't have access to this you can simply use your fingers with some doggy toothpaste on there to get rid of the tartar. Beware, your dog may accidentally bite you! If your adult dog isn't used to the process of getting their teeth brushed yet, start training them by having a routine every single day. Just like bathing, reward them with lots of praise and treats after a successful brushing to help them have a positive association with that activity.

Below are a set of instructions specific to how you should brush the teeth of an adult dog:

1. Buy a doggy toothbrush. These should be readily available at any pet store in your neighborhood. These types of toothbrushes have softer bristles that won't irritate your dog's gums and are built to give you easier access to the teeth that are hard to reach. Larger breeds will require a larger toothbrush and smaller breeds can use a smaller one. As we mentioned before if you don't have a doggy toothbrush readily available you can

use your finger. You can actually buy a product called 'finger brush' that fits on the end of your finger and you can use it as a brush. This gives you better accuracy and precision during the brush compared to an actual toothbrush but you may risk accidentally getting bitten by your dog. Never use a human toothbrush to brush your dog's teeth as the bristles are too hard and could damage your dog's gums, tongue, or the entire mouth.

2. Buy toothpaste that is made for dogs. There should be a wide selection of doggy toothpaste at your local pet store. Never ever use human toothpaste to brush your dog's teeth as our toothpaste typically contains chemicals and fluoride that are very toxic to dogs. Human toothpaste isn't harmful to us since we spit out our toothpaste after each brush but dogs tend to swallow their

toothpaste. Dog toothpaste is also made in different flavors that are appealing to your dog to make the brushing process easier.
3. Start getting your dog comfortable with having your hand near their mouth. When you first begin the brushing session, make sure to go slowly and get your dog used to your hand in their mouth area. It may take some time for an adult dog to get used to being touched there but the more you do it, the more comfortable they will be.
4. Begin the teeth brushing process by letting your lick and try some of the toothpaste. If it is in a flavor that your dog likes, it will make the brushing process more enjoyable for them. It will also help them get used to the taste of the toothpaste.
5. Get your dog used to the actual toothbrush itself by letting him/her sniff or inspect it. Place some toothpaste on the brush and let

your dog taste some off of the toothbrush. Give your dog some praise if they have successfully licked some toothpaste off the brush to help associate this action positively.

6. Now you can gently begin brushing your dog's teeth. Start by brushing the teeth that are easiest to reach like their canines (the longest and biggest teeth). Gently lift up your dog's lip and begin to brush their teeth gently. You can include a family member or friend to help you with this if your dog is having trouble staying still during this. After a few minutes of brushing reward your dog with a treat for his/her good behavior.

7. Once you have brushed all of your dog's teeth, make sure to finish off by brushing the top and bottom surfaces of his/her teeth. Use one hand to hold the top of your dog's muzzle and open his/her mouth. Once your dog's mouth is open, start brushing the bottom

surface of their upper teeth and the upper surface of their bottom teeth.
8. Make sure you make teeth brushing a daily routine as the more often you do it, the more easy it is for your adult dog to get used to it.

Neutering

If you have never owned a dog before then you may not understand the importance of neutering/spaying your dog. If adopted an adult dog, 99% of the time the shelter would have done the neuter/spay surgery already. If for some reason your adult dog is not neutered or spayed, you need to begin the process immediately. Not only will neutering and spaying prevent overpopulation of dogs it also prevents numerous medical issues. Every year, millions of dogs are euthanized because shelters don't have space or resources to take care of them all. By neutering/spaying your own dog, you are playing your part in preventing overpopulation and unnecessary euthanization.

Since neutering is a more important topic for puppies, I will only touch on this subject lightly. Most adult dogs are already neutered/spayed but in the scenario that yours isn't, you will learn all the things you need to know regarding this topic in this chapter.

Neutering and spaying have the same common goal - to prevent dogs from reproducing. Neutering is the surgery for a male dog where he is sterilized so he cannot parent any puppies. Spaying is the surgery for a female dog where she is sterilized so she also cannot parent any puppies. Neutering is a very simple surgery where the stalks of the testicles are cut and then removed from the dog's scrotum. Other benefits to neutering include; lower risk of certain diseases, unwanted behaviors, and socialization problems.

Having your male dog neutered will also prevent your dog from being too territorial. A dog who is very territorial tends to mark places in and outside of your home with their urine as an indication of dominance. When your dog is neutered, they have lowered testosterone levels which will improve unwanted behaviors like marking, aggression, and humping. However, keep in mind that getting your male dog neutered will prevent humping is a myth. A lot of the time your dog humps as a way to exert dominance.

Generally, male dogs can be neutered any time after two months of age but veterinarians advise to wait until your dog hits puberty at six months old. This is a popular time where people get their puppies neutered. Therefore, it is often strange to come across an adult dog who is not already neutered. The process of the surgery is actually very straightforward and the recovery time for male dogs is two weeks.

As we mentioned, neutering and spaying produces the same result in both male and female dogs. The spaying procedure, however, is a lot more invasive than the neutering procedure. In this procedure, your female dog will have her ovaries and uterus removed. This surgery will take more than two weeks for your dog to recover from. However, she will have much better health and other benefits as a result of this surgery. Some benefits include reduced risk of certain illnesses (e.g. mammary gland cancer), no heat period, and no menstruation. Female dogs tend to be in heat every eight months for three weeks at a time. They also don't have menopause so they are able to carry babies for their entire lives until they are spayed. Moreover, female dogs have their periods just like humans and can be extremely messy for your home. Spaying your female dog is a must to prevent mess, smells, and to improve the health of your dog.

Socialization

Understanding what socialization is and why it is important is crucial to owning an adult dog. Most dogs need to be properly socialized between the ages of 2 - 4 months in order for them to have a healthy adulthood. Since you are bringing home your dog as an adult, test out their socialization skills slowly over the course of a few weeks. Socialization is necessary for your dog to get used to the different sounds, sights, and smells of the world from a positive perspective. Since your adult dog likely had a previous owner, you need to start by getting your dog comfortable in their new environment which is your home. Get them comfortable in each room, floor, and outside areas as well. You can then slowly transition them into getting socialized with other people, dogs, places and different situations.

Since your dog has likely come from a different home and you are unsure of their level of socialization, start by testing out what types of situations, places, people, or other animals they are comfortable around. Try to identify situations where your dog appears to be uncomfortable and note those places down. These will be the places that you will start exposing your dog to and positively reinforcing it by making good memories there. Different from puppies where EVERYTHING is new to them, adult dogs typically have a good understanding of common places like the park or the veterinarian. Try to expose your dog to different people and animals and get an understanding of how well socialized they are under those situations. Just the same as noting a place down, start noting down the people or animals that your dog seems uncomfortable with and start focusing on those areas. For example, if your dog is uncomfortable around other dogs to try to set up doggy play dates with other dog parents. Start by having a supervised play date in a comfortable place and get your dog accustomed to other dogs. Always remember to reward with a treat after a successful play date to create a positive association for your dog.

Remember to always continue to take your dog outside their comfort zone during their adulthood. Although they may have been comfortable with a place or a situation during their puppyhood, if they haven't been exposed to it in a while they will forget and become uncomfortable in that situation. Make sure you are constantly taking your dog out to different places and meeting different people. The more situations your dog is exposed to, the less anxious they will be in new situations. If you are adopting your dog straight out of the shelter, consult the staff there and ask questions around your dog's level of socialization skills. They should have a general idea if they are good around other animals, people, and certain places.

Importance of Routine Veterinary Visits

A common misconception of the veterinarian is that you only take your dog there if they are sick or unwell. This is absolutely not true and a responsible dog owner should be taking their dog to the veterinarian for a yearly routine check-up even if nothing is visibly wrong. This is very crucial to your pet's overall health especially if they are in their adulthood or seniorhood.

During the routine visits, the veterinarian will assess how your dog is aging and progressing through life. They will help check for any underlying health conditions that may not be visible to the naked eye. Often times, dogs can have serious issues that aren't noticed by their owners but easily noticed by a veterinarian. It is always much better to spot a problem early so that you are able to correct it or slow the condition down.

Moreover, during general check-up sessions, the veterinarian will always perform a physical examination. This will be a check-up that starts at your dog's nose all the way to the end of their tail. The veterinarian will inspect everything from your dog's mouth, paws, coat, tail, and skin. They will also pay extra attention to your dog's dental health as almost 80% of dogs will be afflicted by dental problems at some point in their life.

By making sure you are bringing your dog to routine check-ups will make sure your veterinarian is keeping tabs on your dog's health. For example, there are vaccines that need to be done every single year and your veterinarian will make sure you are caught up with that so your dog doesn't catch any diseases. In addition, your dog's body is always changing due to age so your veterinarian can help advise the necessary food or diet that your dog needs specific to its stage of life.

Senior dog care taking tips

One population of dogs that are heavily neglected is the senior dogs. Senior dogs have different care requirements compared to adult dogs and puppies. Different breeds of dogs also have different time frames when they are considered senior. For example, larger dogs like the Great Dane are considered to be a senior dog when they are 5 - 6 years old while smaller dogs like Chihuahuas are considered middle-aged at 5 - 6 years old.

So what are some of the things you should expect when your dog begins to age? First of all, your dog may develop arthritis that would slow him/her down. Your dog may not be able to walk or play as often or intensely. He/she will also get tired more easily compared to younger dogs. You may find that your dog will be reluctant in going up and downstairs. If the owner hasn't been properly caring for the dog's dental hygiene, then dental disease becomes a big problem in old age. Statistics actually show that veterinarians can find dental disease in dogs as early as 2 - 3 years of age. If you haven't cared for your dog's mouth, you may find that your senior dog has already lost some teeth.

A lot of the time due to dental disease, your senior dog may be suffering from weight loss. Since their teeth are weakened, your dog may begin to eat less which will cause nutrient deficiency which causes the loss in weight. Senior dogs also frequently suffer from liver disease, kidney disease, and heart disease. All of these above diseases are big contributors to weight loss.

However, some senior dogs may face the opposite problem. Some dogs will become less active due to arthritis or age and become reluctant to exercise or play. This will cause weight gain. Obesity, in general, is a huge problem in the entire dog population but especially significant in the senior dog population. So what are the things we can do to take care of our senior dogs properly?

- Make sure to be scheduling regular visits with your veterinarian. You need to have a bare minimum of one consultation a year when your dog is in seniorhood. It is a lot cheaper to prevent disease than to treat it!
- Get a body evaluation at every appointment. Get your veterinarian to do a complete body evaluation to determine if your dog is at an ideal body weight, overweight or underweight. You may even want to ask your veterinarian to teach you how to evaluate your dog's body at home so you can keep closer tabs.
- Use food as your technique to maintain a healthy body weight for your dog. Since

overweight dogs are at higher risk of heart disease, diabetes, skin disease, and cancer, your veterinarian can help you choose the optimal diet to ensure that all nutrients are being met while maintaining a healthy weight.

- Consider including more fatty acids like DHA and EPA into your dog's diet. These acids have been shown to be extremely effective for dogs that are suffering from mobility issues due to joint diseases like arthritis.
- If your senior dog has heart or kidney disease start considering a special diet. Your veterinarian can recommend the best dog food for your dog based on their condition.
- Continue to take care of your dog's gentle hygiene. Try to have daily brushings in order to keep the tartar at bay. If you aren't able to do so, consider purchasing dental treats or toys that will help your dog clean their teeth.

- Make sure your senior dog is getting exercise. Older dogs are healthiest when they are lean and can maintain healthy muscles and joints. Keep in mind that you have to tailor exercise for your dog based on its individual requirements. If your senior dog is not used to exercise, take baby steps and gradually increase the intensity over time. Make sure to consult a veterinarian for tips on what types of exercises are appropriate for your specific dog.
- Make sure to provide your senior dog with plenty of toys to stay occupied. Senior dogs get bored too so get him toys like food puzzles to help keep him on his toes and his mind fresh.
- Provide your dog with special accommodations depending on their condition. For example, dogs suffering from arthritis would appreciate softer bedding

where they sleep. Ramps can be added into your home when stairs become too difficult. Things like carpeting or rugs will also help your dog walk around your home easier.

Chapter 9

Resolving A Behavioral Problem In Dogs

House soiling is not always a housetraining problem. Often dogs who are perfectly trained will still mess in the home. There are multitudes of reasons for this and any of them may be applicable to your pet, but they will either be categorized as a medical issue or a behavioural problem. It is critically important that the underlying cause is correctly identified if we are to have any success overcoming it. This will require eliminating what does not apply to your dog and taking note of what is triggering the behaviour to occur:

1. The most important issue to rule out is medical. Your animal should visit the veterinarian as soon as you notice the

problem is occurring repeatedly. They will enjoy a comprehensive physical exam, urinalysis, a blood profile test and scrutiny of their medical history. Any abnormalities discovered will prompt further laboratory tests. If the problem is medically related, the vet will discuss a treatment strategy with you. It is possible that medication will prevent further accidents in the house, but you may still need to combine medical treatment with vigilance at home.

2. Should medical causes not be responsible, then you will need to determine the behavioral issue:

- Was your pet ever housetrained properly? In most cases, attempts were made but the process never completed.
- When the problem started, were there any changes in household rules, routines or activities? This may cause animals to begin

marking or suffer a total breakdown of housetraining.

- Has another animal, person or baby joined the household? Often this will trigger insecurity, territorial behaviours or a housetraining memory lapse.
- Is your pet marking or simply urinating? This is easy to identify by the location of the mess. If puddles are found on the floor, then it is urination. If the animal is releasing smaller amounts on horizontal surfaces (such as table legs, furniture or other household objects), then it is marking.
- Is the mess a symptom of separation anxiety? Perhaps the accidents occur when you leave the house or when the animal is locked in a confined area.
- Is the animal displaying signs of submissive urination? In these cases, accidents are triggered by people looming over them, men

speaking too loudly, eye contact, people entering the house, loud noises, thunder or any situation that causes the animal to cower, avoid eye contact, roll over or move away during elimination.

- Does your pet lose control when excited? This is applicable if your animal loses bladder control when you come home, before a walk, when someone visits, at feeding time or any scenario where they become so excited that they are unable to contain themselves.

- Is your dog afraid of going outside? This is evidenced by hesitation at the door and a general disinterest or obvious fear of the outdoors.

- Does your dog only relieve itself on certain surfaces? Some dogs have a preference for carpets, tiles, wooden floors, pebbles, newspapers, puppy mats or another type of surface. Usually these dogs have never been taught to go elsewhere and we often find that their preferred surface is the only one they had available to them in the past.

1. It is important to note that some medications are directly responsible for an increase in bowel and bladder activity. Should your dog be taking medication for another condition, ask your veterinarian if the side effects may be responsible for their house soiling issues. In these cases, it is not your dog's fault at all and the problem will go away when the medication schedule is completed. If your dog is on medication for life, then you will simply need to be more vigilant about taking them outside on a regular basis.

Resolving a Behavioral Problem

Once your veterinarian has ruled out any medical culprits, we need to begin deciphering what the behavioral problem may be. Every time a dog starts eliminating inside, we must to go back to housetraining them, in addition to solving the underlying cause of the issue. We need to stress the importance of identifying the correct problem if we are to be remotely successful. The strategy for a dog suffering separation anxiety is completely different from that used for a fear of going outside. It is absolutely vital that we do not create bigger problems inadvertently, or invite alternative behaviors to manifest instead. If, after several weeks, you are not combating the problem or it is getting worse, call a certified animal behavior expert to help you.

Housetraining

The importance of effective housetraining is paramount. It is simple really; dogs should not soil the house. It smells horrific. It causes stains deep within carpets and wooden floors. It looks terrible when not cleaned up and is a potential hazard that may cause serious injury. People with dogs that are not housetrained tend to end up lonely; friends and family do not enjoy holding their noses for any length of time. Forget about your expensive shoes being ruined by an ill-placed step, worry instead about slipping and breaking your neck!

Has My Dog Been Housetrained at All?

All puppies must be considered untrained. When young, they are unaware of their bodily functions and are unable to control them. As they grow, their ability to 'hold it in' improves. However, they will still be prone to accidents until they reach at least six months of age (sometimes longer). A dog that has continually soiled in the house throughout their life is likely not housetrained. Those that have lived in kennels or who were once outside dogs are also prime candidates. Dogs with an unknown history, usually adopted, often display symptoms of no housetraining. When accidents occur all over the home, even when the door is open to the outside world, a complete housetraining strategy is required.

Was my dog's housetraining not completed?

If your dog only soils occasionally, then this is probably the cause. Those with a tendency to mess during the night or early in the morning, have accidents when not given enough outside opportunities, urinate when left alone, eliminate in rooms that are seldom used or hide their discrepancies from sight have not completed their housetraining. Owners need to go back to basics, begin the housetraining procedure from scratch and make sure that it is done correctly the second time around.

Is My Dog Experiencing a Breakdown in Housetraining?

A once perfectly housetrained dog may suddenly appear to 'forget' their training. This primarily occurs when there is a dramatic change in routine, house rules or when the dynamics in the home change (moving the household or the sudden arrival of a newborn baby, a new spouse, a kitten, another dog or a different animal altogether). Once again, the housetraining process will need to be reinstated.

Solving housetraining problems

In normal circumstances, if given a choice, dogs prefer to eliminate elsewhere. They do not generally do their business where they sleep, play or eat. Rewarding your dog for urinating outside (or your designated area) will entice them to go there, but they still need to be prevented from doing it inside. If not, the smell will continue to attract them and they will not learn the value of disposing waste outside. This is the basis of housetraining and it is important to prevent accidents from occurring in the first place.

Successful housetraining relies on putting the right effort into the program. It is worth the short amount of time it will take to train your dog and will ensure a lifetime of urine-free bliss. There are three reliable housetraining methods to use. Each of them should begin the day your puppy or adopted adult dog arrives in their new home (regardless of how old they are). Before you begin the process, there are some important tips that will help you:

- Equip yourself with rewards such as a high-value treat or toy. Rewarding your dog may also take the form of verbal attention or gentle affection. Whatever you decide to use, be consistent with it whenever your dog gets it right. Food rewards are undeniably the most effective, but you will need to wean the dog off them as they become more reliable at going outside. If you do not do this, you run the risk of having to use them forever. Replace the treats with toys or affection occasionally, at random, so that the dog never knows when to expect them.
- Puppies will make mistakes! So will adult dogs. So will you. This is natural and must be

expected. Do not place any emphasis on mistakes. As pups mature and adults learn, accidents will occur less often and slowly disappear altogether. Obviously, this will only happen if you are consistent with their housetraining throughout the entire process.

- Use the right cleaning products (ammonia-free) when a mess is made. Ammonia enhances the smell of urine and encourages dogs to return there. This is counterproductive to the whole housetraining initiative and will quickly undo all the work you have done. Dishwashing liquid is something that everybody has and it works extremely well.

- Make sure that you do not create a commotion at the scene of a crime. Screaming, smacking and 'shoving their face in it' will only cause distrust of you - encouraging them to hide future accidents in inconvenient places that are hard to find or clean. Believe me, it is decidedly not worth the damage this will do to your relationship or the additional behaviour problems this may cause. It is far more beneficial to the housetraining process, you and your dog if the mess is quietly cleaned while the dog is busy elsewhere.

- Become aware of the alarm signals that indicate elimination is imminent. Your dog will tell you when it needs to go outside and it is up to you to understand this communication. It is unfair to be oblivious of these signs, causing your dog to hold it in until it is forced to make a mistake. When a dog needs to go to its toilet, it will start displaying certain behaviors.

These include:

- Sniffing the ground
- Circling or pacing

- Whining
- Lifting their leg
- Pawing at the ground
- Running to and from the door
- Squatting in a ready position
- Leaving the room

Your dog will need to be taken outside to do its business upon waking every morning and before retiring every night, as well as throughout the day. Take them out as early and as late as possible on a daily basis. In fact, this should be your routine for the duration of their lives.

Regardless of which method you use to housetrain your dog, you should give them every opportunity to go outside. Accompany them to the designated waste area and always reward them for urinating in the right place.

As with newborn babies, young puppies will need to eliminate regularly. They are not able to control their bladders or bowels and it is your job to take them outside, before an accident occurs. A trip to the dog toilet is necessary immediately after certain activities and it is wise to know what they are:

Armed with the knowledge of these tips and including them into your strategy will make housetraining your dog really easy. Regardless of which method you choose to use, it is still advisable to take your dog outside to relieve itself during the day (even in the case of very young puppies). Confinement and elimination mats should only be used at night for the quickest results. Should you need to leave the house for whatever reason, it is best to put your dog either outside or confine them to their crate. That way, they are unable to mess in the house while you are away. If you live in extremely cold or snowy areas, and you will be away for the whole day, you may need to build a bigger confinement area inside for your dog. These scenarios may require the use of elimination mats, but it is still advisable to make a plan for outside elimination. Ensure the area is safe, enclosed, provides ample warm shelter and has fresh water available at all times.

Housetraining outside

The ultimate goal of housetraining is to eventually have your dog go outside of its own accord. This is undoubtedly the best method to use because it teaches them exactly what is required from the outset. It is also the cheapest way to achieve your goal, as well as the easiest (provided you maintain vigilance and consistency at all times).

Helpful tips when housetraining your dog outside

Take your dog outside as frequently as possible. Adult dogs will need to urinate around four times a day, so take them out twice as often. Puppies will need to go more regularly. On average, we recommend hourly trips outside for small pups, a two-hour schedule for those slightly older and a three-hour strategy for pups entering their teenage years. Set the alarm to wake you at night. Twice for tiny pups and once for older puppies.

Remove access to water at night during the housetraining process. If your dog is less than three months of age, allow them a drink on their way outside.

Be sure to notice when your dog is communicating their need to you, usually through circling, sniffing, whining, pawing at the ground, scratching or running to and from the door. This requires an immediate trip outdoors. However, if you take them out often enough, they will seldom need to tell you.

Heed the triggers that cause dogs to dispose of waste. Waking, eating, drinking, playing and new experiences (such as meeting strangers, other dogs or other animals) will require an instant garden visit.

Always go to the same place outside. Dogs will return to where they have been before and it is a good idea to take them where the smell is strongest.

Techniques to Use for Outside Housetraining

When it is time to go outside, call your dog. Use an exciting tone of voice and make the process a fun game to play. Avoid screeching, overuse of the dog's name, wild hand clapping or arm flapping. Remain calm, call the dog and go outside. Do not wait for the dog to come to you first. Just go. The dog will follow you almost always. In extremely rare cases, the dog will simply not come. If this applies to you, then locate the dog and gently put a leash on. Then call the dog once and lead it outside.

Upon arrival at your designated area, allow the dog time to sniff and circle. There is no need to say or do anything at this point. Your dog will urinate automatically after it has gone through the natural process.

Choose one word that you would like to teach your dog to obey for the duration of its life. Keep it short and simple. Most people use 'wee', 'pee' or 'piss', but it can be any word you desire. Say this word once to the dog while it is eliminating. Be quiet and calm, without enticing the dog away from what it is doing. After a while, the dog will associate the word with going to the toilet.

Do not interrupt the dog while it is busy. This is sure to distract them and prevent them from emptying themselves completely. Only deliver the reward once the dog has completed their business. Not as they start or while they are doing it. Afterwards.

Always reward your dog for eliminating at the right place. A food treat, a short walk, a quick game, a toy or calm verbal assurance (such as a quiet 'good dog') is praise enough.

- Once accomplished, return to the house.

www.ingramcontent.com/pod-product-compliance
Lightning Source LLC
LaVergne TN
LVHW020442070526
838199LV00063B/4818